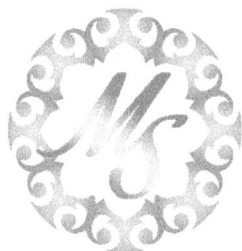

Mhorgan Stephens

i

I Have ITP, But ITP Doesn't Have Me

The Mhorgan Stephens Story

MHORGAN STEPHENS

Cover Design by Juan Gildardo

1st Editing Robin Caldwell

2nd Editing Brenda Bailey BHSB Publishing Company

ISBN:-10:0692665552

ISBN-13:978-0692665558

ACKNOWLEDGMENTS

Before I acknowledge anyone I would like to thank God for always giving me favor and continuing to bless me. I would also like to dedicate this book to my parents, and my sisters, Jassmon and Zyion Stephens. They've been there for me; taking shifts every time I received a treatment to make sure I was okay. I would also like to thank my church, Love Center, for remaining my strong prayer warriors and teaching me that prayer can change anything. I would like to thank Richland Palmetto Children's Hospital for discovering my ITP, also known as **idiopathic thrombocytopenic purpura**, and going above and beyond to educate me about this blood disorder. The loving nurses there continually made sure I had enough arts and crafts to keep me busy. This book is also dedicated to my mentor Yolanda McCutcheon for pushing me to write and showing me that no matter how old you are, you can accomplish and do whatever you set your mind to. I would also love to dedicate this book to all of my friends who helped me stay levelheaded and always made sure I was good. Last but not least, this book is dedicated to anyone dealing with ITP or any blood disorders, and to Lauren Dickerson, who was the first person I met who also had ITP. Thank you for showing me that despite whatever disorder you have, never let that stop you from enjoying life and living it to the fullest. Memories of our time together will forever be in my mind, as well as the lessons you taught me. I will never forget you. Rest in peace, Lauren, and please continue to watch over me. And a special thank-you to Robin Caldwell for making this book come together.

CONTENTS

PROLOGUE

"It's all a mind game." That's what my mother said to me; something that I thought I'd never be able to comprehend or understand. My mother repeated herself: "This is not over for you, Mhorgan. Don't give up. It's all a mind game." What did she mean? I didn't understand the doctor telling me I have **idiopathic thrombocytopenic purpura** or ITP, a chronic disorder, and she's telling me it's all a mind game. What was that supposed to mean?

What is ITP? Well, you're about to find out. My life went from enjoying normal everyday activities to being in a hospital regularly, receiving numerous treatments, and being stuck with needles four to five times a week.
To me, the pain and frustration was anything but a mind game, but as they say, "Mother knows best." At least, I hoped she did.

CHAPTER 1

When I was eight, I moved to Columbia, South Carolina. I was just starting the third grade. I remember it so well, because I absolutely hated my school and everything about Columbia. At least at the time I thought I did, because it was the first major move that I could actually remember. My dad was in the Army so we moved a lot, but for me, Sumter would always be home. Sumter, South Carolina, is where my family and friends lived. We lived in other states, but we always came back to Sumter to visit.

So third grade was coming up, and we had just settled in our new house, and of course, we were going shopping for the new school year. I was happy because this meant I was getting new clothes. What six-year old little girl didn't love new clothes? Well, when I found out my new school had a uniform policy that quickly changed. At first, I was like "Mom, you have to be kidding me," but being the parents of three girls, my parents absolutely loved the idea of uniforms. This meant they saved money, and they always said it would help us "focus" on school more since we were all wearing the same thing.

I finally came to realize they weren't changing their minds, and I quickly got over it. I was fine with wearing khaki pants and navy blue or white shirts. But of course my mom wasn't having that. She wanted me to wear a skirt. *A skirt.* Like an actual skirt that would show my legs. When she made me wear one I was completely devastated.

Growing up I kept getting these weird spots that just appeared all over my body. I went to doctors and even some dermatologists, but they either couldn't find an answer for me or just diagnosed it as eczema. My mom loved to blame it on my not drinking enough water or me being entirely too rough when I played outside. Whatever the case, I had to deal with the fact that I was walking into a new school, where I didn't know anyone and my self-esteem was literally going to be shattered. I just knew everyone would be pointing at the scars on my legs and asking me what happened, and the truth was I didn't have an answer. I had no clue what had happened.

I remember waking up early because I couldn't really sleep. I had excitement about the new school, my nerves were killing me, and then I was sad because I wouldn't be at school with my friends. I woke up the next morning, and I ran into the kitchen to get a glass of "red" Kool-Aid, and intentionally poured it on the skirt I was supposed to wear to school. My dad had already ironed our clothes for school, and placed them out on a chair. I went in the bathroom happy because I knew since my skirt was messed up I would have to wear some pants, right? Yeah, wrong. I came out of the bathroom and tried to cry to my mom about how disappointed I was about not being able to wear my skirt to school and she didn't need to worry because I had some back-up pants on my bed that I could easily throw on. Well, luckily for me, my mom said she had a whole bag full of skirts and she had no problem ironing another one for me. She said next time be careful when drinking your Kool-Aid and kissed me on my forehead and walked out of the room.

"Zyion, Mhorgan, and Jassmon, hurry up and come by the door to take your first day of school picture." Jassmon said, "Mom, do we really have to?" She said, "Yes, because it's your first day in middle school and Zyion and Mhorgan's first day at their school in their uniforms."

"Okay, Mom, please just hurry up because I don't want to be late," said Zyion.

My new school wasn't even three minutes away; it was literally right down the street from my house. If the road had a sidewalk all the way to the school we'd probably walk because that's just how close it was. However, it felt as if we were in the car for hours. Zyion, who is my little sister, was so happy all she did was talk. She said, "Mhorgan, Mhorgan, we're almost closer. Look outside the window, Mhorgan. We're here!" I yelled, "Shut up, Zyion, nobody cares." Of course my mom looked back at me and said, "Mhorgan, that is not how you treat your sister. Now apologize and make sure you watch out for her while y'all are here. Be sure to check on her if you get a chance."

I took a long sigh as the words "Yes ma'am," came out my mouth. Then I grabbed my book bag, opened the door, and prepared myself for what was about to be *the worst* day of my life. My mom walked me into the school and after we dropped my little sister off at her class, we had a conversation on the way to mine. Before I went into my classroom I remember my mom telling me not to worry about anything. "Baby girl, you're going to be just fine. The kids are going to love you, and trust me, nobody is going to be paying attention to those scars on your leg. Stop overreacting and relax. You're beautiful, absolutely beautiful, and don't let anyone here tell you different." I said, "Yes ma'am," taking a deep breath looking down at the floor in the hallway. My mom told me she loved me as she gave me the tightest hug, which made me feel as if I couldn't breathe, because I was all in her shirt. I told her "I love you too," fixing my ponytail and bangs quickly before the teacher got to the door and opened it.

"Hi, you must be Mhorgan," Mrs. Dearmond said, motioning me and my mother to come into the class. I was trying too hard to force a smile on my face, as if I really wanted to be there. She continued, "Well, I'm going to be your English, math, and science teacher. Let me introduce you to everyone. Ladies, I would like for all of you to say hi to Mhorgan." The class of girls shouted, "Hi, Mhorgan!" as they turned and looked at me. It caught me off guard. I was sure it was a mistake—it had to be. Nothing but girls in one class? Oh gosh, I was ready for this nightmare to be over already!! I remember thinking my class was really different and that I kind of liked it. That was the first time I was ever in a class of all girls, and it wasn't just a regular classroom with your typical desks and cubbies, with the white board and teacher's desk in the middle. This classroom had computers for everyone almost like a mini library, except your desk was the place where your computer was. I was extremely excited but tried hard not to show it because I didn't want my mom to leave so soon. After a couple of minutes though she did, and I tried hard to act as if it didn't bother me though it did. I remember sitting down in front of my computer and praying to God that the day went by quickly. A girl next to me said, "You must be new because I never saw you before." I mentioned to her that I was and she told me not to worry, because everybody was nice, "and we all grew up together, so you're the only new one. My name is Sarah. What's yours?" Looking at her I said, "I'm Mhorgan."

"Okay Mhorgan, you can just stay with me today and eat lunch and stuff. I'll introduce you to a lot of my friends." "Okay cool," I said, even though on the inside I was extremely happy I wouldn't have to go through my first day alone. "Oh and by the way, your skirt is really cute," Sarah added. I said thanks, smiling so hard because my mom was actually right. For the rest of the day I actually had fun meeting new people and telling them why I moved and sharing the same interests. Most of all, I was happy that for once, I was happy and gained my self-confidence that day. Since that day I wasn't ashamed of those weird spots that were all over my legs.

School actually went by really fast, and I was excited to get home and just share my story with everyone. My dad made spaghetti that night, and I just gotten out the bathtub, put on my PJs and sat down at the table. "So how was your day?" my dad asked. My oldest sister Jassmon looked as if she didn't want to talk about it. All she said was, "It was okay. I guess I just miss my friends." My youngest sister, Zyion, only in kindergarten, said, "I love my school. I had so much fun! My teacher is cool and we got to play games, color, take a nap, and watch some video on counting. It was cool. There was this song and I'll just sing it for you." Jassmon and I shouted no, we didn't want to hear Zyion sing. My parents both looked at us and said, "That's enough you two." They told us to stop being rude to Zyion. I said "yes, ma'am" to my mom, and Jassmon said "yes, sir" to Dad.

My mom said, "Well Mhorgan, we heard how your sisters' day went; how was yours?"

"Well um, my day was okay," I said, twirling the fork in

my spaghetti just waiting on my mom to ask me more questions. I didn't want to seem too happy because I knew my sister Jassmon hated the fact that we moved and her day didn't go well. So I wanted my mom to know I had a good day but didn't want to say it with a lot of enthusiasm, because I wanted my sister to know I totally agreed with her and didn't want to move either.

"Well I'm glad my beautiful smart daughters had a good day at school," my mom said as we all finished eating our spaghetti and drinking lemonade. "Make sure your homework is signed and leave the papers out for me to sign," she added. "Yes, ma'am," we said as we headed back to our rooms. I just knew that it would be the start of something great. As much as I didn't want to admit it, my mom was right. I was going to love my new school, make friends, and get over wearing a uniform to school because it honestly wasn't that bad. I was going to love this school.

CHAPTER 2

Two years later I was in the fifth grade at the same school. That year I was extremely happy for school to start—primarily because I had the option to wear a uniform or not, and I was finally going to be in a class with both girls and guys.

The night before my first day as a fifth-grader was hectic. After three hours of debating what to wear, my sister finally helped me. She was going to the eighth grade and I was so happy. I just knew my outfit was going to be the best one in the class, because my older sister picked it out for me. I had my blue jeans with a white tank top and pink Aeropostale shirt that looked like the Polo shirts with three buttons. I also had some pink and white Air Force Ones. I just knew my outfit was perfect. I had pink bracelets and white stud earrings, too. The only thing I needed to top everything off was the perfect hairstyle. So of course my mom had just finished braiding my little sister's hair and then it was my turn.

"Okay, Mhorgan, what type of hairstyle do you want?"

"I want the doughnut bun with the swoop bang like you do for Jassmon's hair, Mom."

I HAVE ITP, BUT ITP DOESN'T HAVE ME

Sitting on the floor between my mother's legs, I turned my head and looked at her face, because I just knew she was going to say no. But surprisingly she said, "Okay, Mhorgan, you better not mess your hair up when I do it; and take care of it." I said, "Yes ma'am."

I usually didn't wake up for school until six and my sister woke up at five in the morning. I was so happy I woke up at five, too. This was it. My last year in elementary school. I had a lot of friends and we were finally going to be   the   big   kids   in   school.

People were literally going to be looking up to us. I took my time to make sure my jeans and shirt were ironed with no wrinkles. I made sure I had a white and pink ribbon to tie around my bun. My earrings matched my necklace, which matched my shirt that matched my shoes. My sister made sure to mention to me that I was a big girl so all of my outfits needed to look like hers. I needed to start acting like a girl because the guys don't like a girl who acts like a tomboy, she said. Also I started modeling, and I couldn't wait to brag about it to the people and kids at school.

The first day of school was great; it felt like a reunion with everyone and we all caught up on things. It was fun seeing how a lot of people changed and grew up a little over the summer. My class was amazing. I loved everything about the teachers and people in the class. For once, I actually had guys in my class after what seemed to be forever of having all-girl classes. I felt normal again. A couple of weeks passed by and we got a new student. His name was Brian. Oh my gosh! Brian was so cute. He had hazel eyes and short brown curly hair. His smile was perfect. Every girl in my class had a huge crush on him, including me.

My teacher Ms. Hunter welcomed Brian to come sit down at the desk right beside mine. She said, "Mhorgan, please help Brian get situated and fill him in on some things we've been talking about during our break time."

"Yes, Ms. Hunter," I said, jumping up and down on the inside. Break time finally came around and I was like, "Hey Brian, I'm Mhorgan. I guess you can follow me around all day and I'll show you where the library and stuff is if you want."

"Okay cool," said Brian.

"Okay cool," I said, trying so hard not to smile and let him know I had this huge crush on him. We were working in groups of two for a project that we wouldn't start until the next day. Ms. Hunter had already paired us up so we could be aware of our partners.

The next day I made sure to wear this cute striped dress with some sandals and this pearl necklace. Brian and I were working on our project, and he was asking me something I honestly can't remember. I was daydreaming about how perfect he was. I just remember smiling and constantly pushing my bangs out of my face. He was so cute. This was actually the first time we got to have alone time together. Even though technically it wasn't but in my head it was; I was literally the luckiest girl in the classroom. I knew the other girls were livid and I loved it. But the more I realized Brian started to actually pay me attention as in looking me in my face and smile, I got really nervous. It was like I had butterflies in my stomach. What was this feeling? I think I was in love. He was just so gorgeous. His eyes, smile, and even cologne smelled like heaven. I got so distracted I actually bumped my arm on the desk. It didn't hurt though. A couple of minutes later I saw girls pointing at me whispering, and some started laughing. Of course I just figured they were jealous I was working with Brian and they weren't. Then dudes even started doing it so, I thought maybe they're just *hating* like my sister would say. But when I saw Brian's face change and he asked if I was okay, I became really, really confused. That's when Ms. Hunter asked me to step outside for a second. I said, "Yes, ma'am." I was kind of happy to leave because I felt humiliated, like I was a laughingstock. Everyone was laughing and posing like I was a joke, and I couldn't understand what was funny. On the other hand I was scared. *Did I do something? Was I about to get in trouble? Did I fail that vocabulary test we took last week?*

Finally outside Ms. Hunter looked at me and closed the door. "Is there something you'd like to tell me?" I think that's the most rhetorical question someone could ask. Knowing this is the same question my parents usually asked before I always get in trouble, I simply said, "No, Ms. Hunter." Shaking my head as if to say everything's perfect. Smiling as if I was really concerned I asked, "Is there something that you wanted to know?" Ms. Hunter took a deep breath and lowered her voice; speaking in a softer tone that was sincere and said, "Mhorgan, it's okay. You can tell me anything at all. You won't get in trouble. Is everything at home okay? Has anyone been hurting you?"

Totally shocked and freaked out, I tell her no and that I'm fine. "I'm perfect; why do you ask?" Ms. Hunter looked down at my arm then back at me. She pointed at my arm, and asked, "Well if nothing's wrong, then how did you get that?" I just laughed a little and said, "Oh, I just bumped my arm on the desk, Ms. Hunter. It's no big deal."

"Mhorgan, your arm has a huge knot on it."

I immediately looked down at my arm and panicked. That was not the same arm I looked at when I bumped it on the desk earlier. Before it was like a mini bruise but a little darker purple. I figured I just bumped it harder than I thought. But I didn't pay it any mind because of course Brian and I had a project to do, and I really wanted to get my work done. Okay, well maybe I just wanted to sit there and look pretty in front of Brian. But it didn't matter because either way I wasn't concerned with the small bruise on my arm. But now that I was outside the classroom with Ms. Hunter, I was kind of worried because it looked like a small anthill on my left arm. I had no clue where it came from and how it came from a small bump on the desk. Ms. Hunter seemed relieved knowing it came from a small bump on the desk, and I assured her it wasn't hurting so she sent me to the nurse to get some ice.

I came back, first kind of nervous at what everyone would say, but also kind of happy I finally realized why people were looking and laughing. Brian saw the ice and asked if I was okay and to make sure I wasn't in pain. Though I knew there was nothing he could do about it, I didn't care. I loved every bit of attention that he was giving me. He told me he would stay inside with me during recess or sit outside to keep me company since the nurse and teachers wouldn't let me play. I almost fainted because I was so flabbergasted. I didn't even know what to say. Was this his way of asking me on a date? Even though I was only in fifth grade I had seen a lot of movies and shows about people taking each other on dates, and my sister talked about them with her friends over the phone. So I said, "Okay cool. It's a date." Brian looked at me with a shocked smiled and said okay cool.

Finally the recess bell rang and everybody ran outside toward the track to meet up and socialize. Brian and I walked outside the school, taking our time, in no rush. We sat at the table right in front of the track, and of course, my arm still had the ice pack on it. I was icing my arm so long I thought it would fall off.

The teachers were all standing up in a circle doing what my friends and I call "gossiping" about old people stuff. That's when my teacher called me to come over to her. She told me to explain to the teachers what I did in class and then wanted me to show them. It had been at least two hours after I bumped my arm, and I'm not exaggerating: my arm was almost the size of a softball or tennis ball! The lump just looked bigger and it was purple. The ice didn't seem to be much help. All of the teachers were looking in amazement and terrified. The look on their faces was as if they'd seen a science project that's really interesting but at the same time very weird. They were not sure if they should be curious or scared. I felt like it was show and tell for the rest of the day, and my arm was what everybody wanted to see. In a weird way a lot of people were so fascinated that I had that huge knot on my arm from simply bumping it on a desk.

After school I got in the car excited because I was on the way to modeling practice. My modeling school was right down the street and I remember getting out and running inside because I was late, and I didn't want to miss my turn walking down the runway. My mom usually waited in the parents' room until practice was over, which was only an hour. But I couldn't even get into practice for 10 minutes until the other girls started freaking out asking me what happened to my arm. That's when my modeling director took me outside the room to show my mom and talk to her.

At first my mom was furious. She had no clue what happened to me and when. Being only eight, I simply forgot to mention it to her and I didn't think it was a big deal. My mom is a nurse so looking at the knot and bruise on my arm she assumed it was broken and immediately called the doctor. She was freaking out about my teacher not telling her or calling her, and I simply explained it wasn't the school's fault because I told her not to call. My mom was still not happy with my answer as to why they never contacted her. She stuck her index finger up at me, motioning me to hush and she talked to my doctor, explaining what happened and that she was bringing me over immediately.

I was sad because I really wanted to finish my modeling practice and I felt perfectly normal. But my mom and modeling director assured me I could miss this practice and go to the next one because my health was way more important. I went to the doctor. By the time I arrived, my mother had already contacted my father. The doctor of course wanted to draw blood. That didn't sit too well with me because I really didn't care much for needles. However, I wasn't like my older sister, and it wasn't necessary for me to have eight people holding me down to draw my blood or give me a shot. I wasn't crazy about the idea of having somebody put a needle in my arm, but if that meant I would find out what was wrong I was okay with that. I remember waiting about 30 minutes after my blood was drawn, though it felt like hours. I could tell something was wrong and his exact words were: "I've already called the emergency room, they're waiting on her. Either I can call an ambulance for her or you can drive her but she needs to rush there immediately. Her platelets are 2,000."

I'll never forget that look on my mother's face. It was as if someone said somebody died or like someone stabbed her with a knife. I felt like I was in a movie and everything around me just stopped.

What's going on? Why am I going to the hospital? What

happened? Mom, why are you about to cry? Mom, what does the doctor mean? What are platelets? These are all questions I asked but couldn't get any answers to. You see, I'm so used to doctors saying things, and then my mom interpreting them for me. She would break down the words so I could understand.

This time was different. When we finally got to the ER, they immediately took me back, and I had to put on a hospital gown, and people started attaching this machine to me, drawing more of my blood. After spending hours in the room—which was cramped because it held me, my mom, father, and grandma—the doctor came in and said, "She doesn't have leukemia; however, it is ITP. We will be admitting her overnight and giving her some treatments to boost her platelets."

At this point my mom is in tears, crying in her chair as if she'd heard the worst thing ever. My dad had never been an emotional person, but that day I looked into his eyes, and I could see his pain. However, I couldn't feel it.

CHAPTER 3

What is ITP

"What is ITP?" I asked the doctor. "What does this mean? Why am I in the hospital for it?"

The doctor turned around and looked at me, pulled a chair up to the bed, and sat down. He said, "ITP is a fairly common blood disorder that both children and adults can develop."

There are two forms of ITP: **Acute thrombocytopenic purpura.** This usually affects young children, ages 2 to 6 years old. The symptoms may follow a viral illness, such as chickenpox. Acute ITP usually starts suddenly and the symptoms usually disappear in less than six months, often within a few weeks. Treatment is often not needed. The disorder usually does not recur. Acute ITP is the most common form of the disorder. **Chronic thrombocytopenic purpura** is the onset of the disorder, which can happen at any age, and the symptoms can last a minimum of six months, several years, or a lifetime. Adults have this form more often than children do, but it does affect adolescents. Females have it more often than males.

Chronic ITP can recur often and requires continual follow-up care with a blood specialist, which is a hematologist. The normal platelet count is in the range of 150,000 to 450,000. With ITP, the platelet count is less than 100,000. By the time significant bleeding occurs, you may have a platelet count of less than 10,000. The lower the platelet count, the greater the risk of bleeding.

"So for your platelet count to be 2,000, that's extremely low," he said.

My next question was, "Okay, how did I get ITP?" That's when Dr. Brown said, "The cause of ITP is unknown, but the disease involves two processes: the destruction of existing platelets and inadequate production of platelets to make up for those being destroyed." After he said that, I was trying not to ask a lot of questions, especially what exactly were platelets?

Platelets are small, disc-shaped cell-like particles that are made in the bone marrow by cells called megakaryocytes and circulate through the bloodstream. Platelets help stop bleeding by forming clots when blood vessels are damaged. Typically, a platelet is removed from the bloodstream after seven to ten days. But in an adult patient with ITP, antibodies attack platelets, so they are removed and destroyed much sooner than that—even as soon as a few hours after they enter the bloodstream. Antibodies may also attack the megakaryocytes, which may prevent these cells from making as many platelets as they typically would have.

"Soooo...I have ITP? Is that the real name of it, Dr. Brown?"

Dr. Brown looked at me and said, "Well no, Mhorgan. The real name of it is **idiopathic thrombocytopenic purpura. Also sometimes called** immune

thrombocytopenic purpura or simply, immune thrombocytopenia. **Thrombocytopenia** means a decreased number of platelets in the blood.

"**Purpura** refers to the purple discoloration of the skin, as with a bruise," he explained.

I asked my doctor one last question. "Well, how are you sure that I have ITP? What makes you think you're right?"

Dr. Brown laughed and said I had a lot of questions for an eight-year-old, that I had definitely asked more than most of his other patients who had been diagnosed with ITP. I just simply smiled and said well of course that's what makes me different.

Dr. Brown continued on to say the symptoms of ITP are related to increased bleeding. However, each person may experience symptoms differently. Symptoms may include:

The purple color of the skin after blood has "leaked" under it. A bruise is blood under the skin.

People with ITP may have large bruises from no known injuries. Bruises can appear at the joints of elbows and knees just from movement.

Tiny red dots under the skin that are a result of very small bleeds

Nosebleeds.

Bleeding in the mouth and/or in and around the gums.

Heavy menstrual periods.

Blood in the vomit, urine, or stool.

Bleeding in the head. (This is the most dangerous symptom of ITP. Any head injury that occurs when there are not enough platelets to stop the bleeding can be life threatening.)

After hearing a list of just some of the symptoms I was shocked. More than half of those I had. The constant nosebleeds my parents and I assumed were from being overheated easily, and when I got overheated my nose just bled. My gums bled often but my mom and I assumed maybe it was because I was brushing too rough.

This explained the bruises I kept getting. Also the spots I had weren't eczema they were simply symptoms of ITP.

This was all slowly but surely starting to make sense to me. Because at this time, even though I was only eight, I had a lot of family members in the medical field, and with my mother being a nurse, and me making good grades I was pretty smart for my age. I could also understand a lot when it came to the body.

Looking my mom and dad in their eyes I just simply smiled, and said, "It's going to be okay. Don't worry, God's got this." I think it really shocked everyone in the room, especially the doctor, because they weren't expecting it. But I just knew I had to stay strong and fight.

CHAPTER 4

It's funny how your life can literally change so fast and you have no control over it. Here I was just being a normal sassy, funny, talkative outgoing girl one day, who simply bumped her arm on a desk, to being in the hospital by the end of the day diagnosed with some blood disorder I never knew of or heard anything about.

At the time I was only eight years old but it didn't even matter. All my life I was raised on building my own relationship with God, keeping my faith strong, and being taught to never give up when life gets tough. I grew up in the church, and I was taught how to pray for myself; and whenever something went wrong and I felt hopeless, pray because God would always be there even when it feels like no one else was. So at that moment, I realized that my mindset had to change. I knew nothing about ITP, except for what the doctor just told me. My point was simply this: People are diagnosed with disorders, disabilities, and cancers every day. People are told that they didn't get the job they wanted, or the part for the commercial or movie they were trying for every day. But if we all stopped and gave up everything when we make one mistake or something doesn't go our way, then we'd all be failures and accomplish nothing.

No one in this world is perfect. We all have our flaws and success in life comes when you simply refuse to give up. When you have determination and goals, then obstacles, failure, and loss only act as motivation.

So I had to ask myself, what makes today so different from yesterday? Just because the doctors came and diagnosed me with something didn't mean I had to give up on life. Even though in a matter of hours my life took a dramatic turn, I still felt the same. The reality is we're all humans and make mistakes. Sometimes the doctors could be wrong. Not saying that to put them down, but I say that to say stop letting information and people determine your fate and how you're going to live your life.

I respected the doctors and their treatment decisions to help my ITP, but I didn't get depressed or sad when I was first diagnosed because 1.) I was too young and blessed to be stressed; 2.) I knew God had the last say; and 3.) I felt completely normal, which was the most frustrating part for me. How could I feel fine but have been diagnosed with a serious blood disorder? I suppose this really worked in my favor because it helped me keep my faith strong.

The first thing I tried to do after my parents pulled themselves together was use their phone to research ITP; after maybe an hour or two of research, I became very frustrated because it seemed like all the information started to repeat itself. Almost like I came to a dead end. There wasn't a lot of information out on ITP or blogs for it. This made me think about beginning my own blog for kids with ITP, because I thought it'd be cool for kids with ITP or any blood disorder to have a website or blog where you can discuss how you're feeling and what you're going through with others just like you. This definitely was a goal and dream I hoped to accomplish.

My sisters helped me stay leveled throughout my treatments because they cared, of course, and they were worried about my health. But that didn't really change our relationship. We'd still argue over clothes or shoes but they knew the perfect times to do it.

Having this blood disorder wasn't just affecting me, even though it was my life and my body, it really affected the people around me as well. At first, going through the treatments didn't bother me because I kept my mind off of it by doing arts and crafts like coloring, painting, puzzles, making pillows, just about any and everything you could think of, honestly. Any hands-on activities that seemed fun, I gave a try. Usually my mom would be sitting on a chair right next to the bed or sometimes she'd lie in the hospital bed with me while I received my treatments. She'd constantly remind me, "You got this, Mhorgan. It's all a mind game; stay focused." Doing the different activities really helped get my mind off of what was going on right beside me. Not feeding into the needles and the 24/7 care I received helped me get through it.

Within the first year of my diagnosis, I had visited the doctor and hospital more than I had ever done in my life. I constantly battled with my platelets coming up from 2,000 to 7,000 to 20,000 and then back down. It seemed like nothing would work. It was so frustrating to start a treatment that actually seemed to work, only to use it a few rounds later and realize your body is now immune to it so you have to find another treatment and restart the whole process. I felt like I was on a roller coaster constantly taking loops and turns. However, it was okay because I still got to go to school often, and hang out with my friends.

I HAVE ITP, BUT ITP DOESN'T HAVE ME

CHAPTER 5

During the middle of the school year some girlfriends and I were on the bus discussing how their periods had started already, because I was complaining about having cramps. They kept saying, "Join the club, Mhorgan. Your period is coming." They shared all of their stories about how theirs came as if this was the most exciting thing in the world. Of course, I laughed it off and said, "Yeah, whatever. That's crazy, my period isn't coming; I think I'm just sick or something. Later that night my period came, and I remember yelling and calling my mom because I was not sure what to do. I remember her saying it's okay that it was just my menstrual cycle and every female has one. I took a shower, put on some PJs, and she gave me a pad. Not even thirty minutes later I came in her room to ask for another one so I could change. My mom was on the phone with my aunt and said, "What?"

"No, Mhorgan, I just gave you one. You don't change every thirty minutes."

I cried as blood ran down my leg, saying, "No, Mom, I need another one now!" She jumped up and in shock started freaking out because my menstrual flow was heavy. She tried tampons and a pad and I still managed to bleed through. My period was so heavy I had to go to the ER the next day.

I HAVE ITP, BUT ITP DOESN'T HAVE ME

At first the doctors just said don't worry, because a heavy menstrual period is common, especially because I had ITP. I constantly had to get up and run to the bathroom to change. It felt as if every time I stood up a bunch of blood just gushed down. That was so scary.

The doctors didn't really start doing anything about my periods until I started to clot. My longest period lasted for nine months straight. The doctors were in so much disbelief. After the nine months I would get a period for a few weeks. Then it would start again and last for months at a time. Eventually I prepared myself to live with my just bleeding for the rest of my life. The doctors worked hard trying to find a treatment that would help stop some of the bleedings, which meant more hospital treatments for me. During this time I had the wonderful opportunity to meet a girl named Lauren, who had been diagnosed with ITP just like me. Except hers had become worse than mine, and she was in the intensive care unit (ICU). My mom met her grandmother while she was out of the room, walking down the hall. She asked me to pray for her. Before meeting Lauren I prayed for other kids periodically, simply because through me praying for them I knew it did nothing but make me stronger—and healed me. So of course I said yes, because at the time even at a young age I understood prayer could help change a lot of things. After praying for Lauren, we exchanged numbers, and she and I became close, good friends. We would have movie nights or I would bring her gifts, and she'd give me gifts. We instantly clicked.

It was amazing knowing that other kids your age understand you and are going through the same thing you're going through. Lauren was one of the sweetest most beautiful people I've ever met. She taught me how to keep your faith high and spirits up at all times. She really helped me realize to be grateful for what you have and everything in your life both the good and bad. There is always someone who has it worse than you so always be grateful. Lauren simply had *HOPE*. It didn't matter what obstacles she went through, you'd never be able to tell by her facial expression. Every time you saw her she had a smile that'd cheer you up and warm your heart. No matter how she felt she stayed positive.

ITP really gave me a new perspective and outlook on life simply because it taught me that even though I have ITP, ITP *DIDN'T* have me. One of the gifts Lauren gave me, which I still have to this day, was a white shirt that read, "Lifting Up Lauren." It also had a scripture on the back, for which I will forever cherish and be grateful.

Lauren had one wish. At the time I was still modeling and was going to Orlando, Florida, for a showcase. She simply asked me to wear her shirt and take a picture in it if I went to Disney World. Of course I promised Lauren I would and gave her one last hug—not realizing that would be the last time Lauren and I would ever talk.

I HAVE ITP, BUT ITP DOESN'T HAVE ME

CHAPTER 6

The summer leading into my sixth-grade year my ITP was at a decent point. I was able to keep my platelets at a steady 50,000 and a little below—which technically wasn't too good. If I were in a trauma accident my platelets would have to be at least 75,000 for them to even operate on me. By the third month of my sixth-grade year, I actually found myself homebound and undergoing chemotherapy. Going through chemo was one of the toughest treatments I had to experience simply because it truly did make me feel awful. No matter how hard I would try to force a smile on my face or be that sassy little girl, there were some days I couldn't even get out the bed. I remember lying in the hospital bed one night asking my mom about Lauren. I knew normally when I was in the hospital she was there too, about three doors down. I figured it would have been a perfect night to watch a movie together while we both got our treatments. Honestly, I knew seeing her would automatically put me in a better mood and cheer me up. We called her grandma and had heard Lauren passed away a couple weeks earlier. That was the first time I felt that type of pain. It was indescribable pain that I didn't even know you could have. I was hurt. I felt like I let her down.

She never even got to see the picture I took in her shirt at Disney. I didn't give it to her because I really wanted to put it in the prettiest frame I could find. She saw more potential in me than I thought I had. Lauren said I was a star in her eyes no matter what happened. She was truly my number one fan. She had so much hope for me and believed I would be destined for greatness. That night I felt as if a part of me had left. I lost a friend, a true friend to the same blood disorder that I had. I didn't understand. This was a major wake-up call for me. For the first time I finally understood this *wasn't* a game. It was serious. This disorder, this disease, had the power to take my life away. It took my best friend and so many other innocent people. There's no cure for ITP, which made everything ten times worse.

Going through chemo was not only tough because of the treatment but simply because for the first time I wanted to give up. To me there was no point. I just didn't understand—I couldn't. *Why? Why Lauren? Why me?* I didn't want to have it anymore. I didn't want to deal with this stupid thing anymore. I felt like just giving up; I was tired mentally and physically. Tired of the treatments, tired of going on this roller coaster with ITP and tired of simply being tired. Having to basically isolate yourself from friends, family, activities, and the outside world was one of the most challenging things ever. I was held captive in my own body. Wearing a mask and having people look at you like some creature because you couldn't afford to be sick made me feel inhuman. Slowly the same energetic, always smiling, loud positive girl began to change. I not only began doubting myself but God as well. I felt as if I had no purpose in life and didn't belong. I was sick of being isolated and cut off from society. Sick of being tired, sick of hurting, sick of being poked daily by the needles who fiend for my blood like vampires, sick of having different medications entering my body like I was some test animal. I felt as if no one understood. Nobody truly felt how I did, and to be honest that was simply because no one really did. With all these emotions just scrambling through my mind I found myself not only getting depressed but also just giving up. The aftermath of me doing this led to my body getting sicker. Being surrounded by kids my age with the same disorder and some in way worse conditions—and some even dying—was absolutely heartbreaking. The most disappointing thing was I finally realized I had simply lost hope. I was tired of being sick. I was tired of having to sleep at the hospital; tired of staying home because I couldn't go to school; tired of seeing doctors and nurses, IV's; and tired of dealing with this sickness. I was so tired of feeling normal, or what seemed to be normal, only to have the doctors order another treatment and say my platelets were low. I just wanted everything to go away. I remember I would cry myself to sleep. I'd often pray and ask God, why me? *What did I ever do? Why am I being punished?* I remember telling my mom I just want to go to school, I want to hang out with my friends, and I want to be a model again. I didn't want to keep watching my friends enjoy themselves through social media. I didn't want any more notes or letters about how they miss me and can't wait to see me soon.

I didn't want anyone to have sympathy for me. I wanted to cheer, go shopping, hang outside with my friends. Have sleepovers. I really just wanted my life back. The more I started to realize how much my life changed and dwelled on the past and started thinking negatively, I realized it wasn't doing me any good. At the end of the day, I was still sick and, if anything, worse than I was before.

I remember some nights coming home after my chemo treatments and falling asleep and waking up with chills or fevers, feeling as if I had to puke. My body aching in pain, just really sore. I could barely get out of bed. It was scary. This disorder. This very thing that seemed to turn my life upside down was like a silent killer. That's when my mother had my uncle, who is also my bishop, pray over this pink bandana. He anointed it with oil and my mother gave me two cornrows in my head before tying the scarf over it. We prayed and prayed that I wouldn't lose my hair, because for me, losing my hair would have been the icing on the cake.

That bandana symbolized a lot for me. Every day through my chemo I wore the bandana. For me it was just a reminder of how much support I was getting from my family.

Every time I thought about the bandanna it made me remember to keep fighting because I was a soldier and I had this. As days went by, and the more I received treatment, I realized there was so much going on. There was so much I had to deal with.

It's as if no one understood. Once I realized this, it really started to not only take effect on me but also my sisters and family. I also realized I had to change.

My little sister turned to food as a way to vent and started to gain weight. That was her way of dealing with everything. My oldest sister's grades started to fall, because she had trouble focusing. They were so worried about me they forgot about themselves. They just wanted to make sure their sister was okay. They didn't care if that meant they got no sleep, and stayed up during the night making sure I wasn't having any side effects from my medicine, or always had crafts to do, or took all my medicine. They did whatever it took just to make sure I was going to be okay. The moment I realized that this was affecting more people than just me, I realized it was time to pull myself together.

I had felt sorry for myself long enough and it obviously wasn't doing me any good. I told myself snap out of it. Get yourself together.

I finally understood what my mom meant when she said, "Mhorgan, pull yourself together. It's all a mind game." I realized your mind can have you think your disorder, disability, sickness, or whatever you're going through is huge and horrible when in reality, it's not that bad. The moment I decided to stop thinking negatively and looking for the worst outcomes, I realized I started to become better.

I refuse to even let my mind go there when I'm not feeling great. I refuse to let my mind make me think something that is that bad. Chemo was a long and tiring process. When my mom said, "It's all a mind game," she didn't mean it literally. It doesn't mean if you think positive your disorder, illness, or disability will be gone, and your life is back to normal. It simply means if you can learn how to adjust and train your mind to be more positive and focus on positivity rather than negativity, you'll realize it's less stressful and easier to deal with your situation.

CHAPTER 7

I knew my mother had a lot going on. Being the mother of a child with ITP simply wasn't easy, because that meant that everything else in life wasn't going to stop.

A NOTE FROM MY MOM: I was very excited when I heard that Mhorgan decided to tell her story. I said finally everyone would get to know the young lady that God has entrusted her father and me with, and know the true meaning behind her drive.

When I found out that Mhorgan had ITP, I never imagined writing about my feelings. As a strong believer in God, for the first time, I remember asking, *"Where are you now?"* Yes, as a Christian, I questioned him.

The families that we met at the time had children who were extremely sick and were receiving treatments. To be honest, as a parent, how do you know your child is going to be okay? As a nurse, knowing the lights of the children around her were dimming, how do you talk to your sick child? Truth is, I didn't tell her—she told me.

Mhorgan woke up one night in the hospital and said,

"Mom, God told me as I began to pray for other kids, he would heal me." That's when I knew God never left us. My pastor brought oil from the church and the scarf we had on Mhorgan's head was prayed over, and she then began her daily devotion in her own way. Even when she was too sick to barely move. We would put the mask on her and lay her in the very back of the church. After the preaching was over, we would be the first to leave. The way her body was set up we couldn't afford to take any chances with her since her immune system was so weak. I literally shut everything down around her, so I could focus more on her getting better. Slowly but surely Mhorgan began to walk around with the activity leader during the day, and play with the kids she was allowed to play with; and she would always whisper a little prayer. Within two days, Mhorgan was able to go home. It was at this time I learned it may have become my journey but it was just the beginning of her fight.

***

Mom was right. After I was released from the hospital, I realized that this was only the beginning of my fight. Though I had been dealing with ITP for over a year and remained strong, I realized that this was only the beginning. Forget being in and out of the hospital and at the children's clinic four to five times a week; I realized I wasn't really fighting like I should have fought. Yeah, ITP had its good days and bad days, and of course I was strong enough to get through them. But what about everyone else?

When I left the hospital after chemo, there was something about that particular visit that made it different. I couldn't understand the question, *"Why am I so stuck on this?"* I'll never forget walking out of the hospital on the way to the car and I met this guy outside. He was crying and I had my bear in one arm and was in the wheelchair with my parents behind me. He stopped us and said,

"Thank God your child is going home today. She might still be sick, but my little angel lost her fight today when God called her home this morning. She was only three years old." His words will never be deleted out of my mind. Looking into the man's face, even though I was still young, I really felt his pain and sorrow. On that day I also realized that life is a blessing.

So many times we take the smallest things for granted and often don't even realize the worth or value of it until it's gone. Despite feeling under the weather, I knew I was on a mission. There was a goal to complete, and I refused to stop until it was finished. My main focus at that point was making my first website. I called it KidswithITP.com. I really invested a lot of time and effort into it. I remember staying up for two days straight just doing research. Even though it was really hard to find good valid information about ITP, I knew that some way, somehow, I was going to find it. Indeed I did. After I found my research I remembered that I always wanted to have a blog. So I got my diary, where I wrote all of my encounters with the treatments I went through, and put the blog together. I had pictures and contact information. I was extremely proud of myself because it took me three-and-a-half, almost four whole weeks to do it. The best part was that I did it by myself. While I could have been coloring or watching TV or something along those lines, I chose to work on my website. It may not have been the best website or maybe even the most complex website, but at least I could say, "I did it!" My website wasn't intended to have all the fancy medical terms or even the best gadgets. The purpose was just to let others know, especially kids who were dealing with it, that they weren't alone. And while I'm not a doctor, I still researched to gather information to help educate people a little more about the disorder. I made sure to have websites they could visit if they really wanted to go more into detail about ITP. The blog was really just for people to see how I felt, read about my encounter with the medicines, and allow them to live their own stories. About one month after my website had been up, and my mother actually saw people were interacting with it, she went downtown to get me my own business license. This meant that my dream of having a foundation to help others was coming true. That's when the Kids with ITP Mhorgan Stephens Foundation came alive.

Since then, I've gone to the hospital with candy bags, toys, presents, books, really just about anything you could think of to take to the floor of kids with blood disorders at the hospitals. Of course, I still had lots of things left and those I took down to the clinic. I tried to make sure that on every holiday or special occasion, I was at the hospital giving them something. The main reason is because I knew how I felt being a kid stuck in the clinic or hospital on a special holiday. Even though we had adults who really tried their best to make us feel at home and happy, it wasn't the same as having an actual kid my age doing that. It was just nice to know that there were more than adults who cared. I loved getting to meet the kids and being able to play with them or giving them their gifts. For me, it not only helped get my mind off what was going on, but it made me feel amazing on the inside. I remember reminding children to always stay strong and even though they have that disorder, cancer, or illness, that does not have to stop them from living and accomplishing their dreams. I constantly reminded them to stay positive, humble, and never give up. I always left them saying this: "Don't let the doctor's report or what they say discourage you, because at the end of the day we're all human. Just like you can be diagnosed with something, you can also beat it. Or in my case live your life and try your best to not let it affect you."

CHAPTER 8

I was so grateful to have such a supportive family and friends who stood behind me and helped all my visions come alive. One of the toughest things for me through the chemo was having to wear a mask because my immune system was so weak—going out in public or different places and feeling people stare at me as if I was some type of creature. To me it didn't bother me that they constantly looked at me; I think it was the fact that I knew they were so quick to make assumptions, which were extremely wrong. But after a few times I quickly got used to it and learned to just ignore it. When I was finally able to come back to school, sixth grade was almost over, and I basically didn't know anyone because I was gone for most of it. However, when I came back to school, so many people knew *me*, it was crazy. Apparently my story about receiving chemo and what I was going through got around and surprisingly the support and words of encouragement, not only from my teachers but also my classmates and whole school, was overwhelming at first; but I was so thankful for all of it.

I HAVE ITP, BUT ITP DOESN'T HAVE ME

At first I couldn't find a normal locker like my other classmates because we could not risk books falling on my head or me getting pushed and shoved because everyone was in a rush. So my locker buddy was my assistant principal because I kept my stuff in her office. I quickly adjusted to school and loved every moment of it. Making friends and going to class was amazing. It was good being able to feel like a normal kid for once and not worry about the doctors. For the last three or four months of my sixth grade year I enjoyed every moment and even had the courage to try out for the cheer team. By the end of the year, I made the cheer team and was extremely happy to be a seventh-grader and looked forward to the next year. Making the cheerleading team was huge for me because it was just confirmation for me to know that despite what people say you can't do, they cannot determine your fate and be the last word.

Seventh grade started off great. I wish I could say that I ended up getting rid of ITP and never had any more problems and was finally able to be normal—but that's far from the truth. Being that I was at school and people did get sick and since we were still young, a lot of kids didn't follow the proper methods for killing germs. Therefore I was constantly sick. Thankfully, I was finally homebound, which came in handy because it still allowed me to interact with my friends, but also let me get my school work and everything caught up. Cheering with my friends was so much fun. Even though I couldn't do stunts because it was a huge safety risk for me, I was able to do everything else. I loved all the attention that came with being a cheerleader. The sixth-graders actually looked up to me and everyone else.

Every Monday there was a doctor's appointment for me, and that wasn't including my days of being sick or unexpected medical events. After I was able to get used to this, the rest of my year was great. Something I think is important to know is that being *normal* is really boring. We all have flaws or things that might pop up in life like a disorder in my case or whatever it may be. However, it's vital and extremely important to embrace those things because that's what makes us important and unique. Once I accepted this. everything seemed to go much better.

Toward the end of the year we had health science, which the school taught every year. That year my teacher was talking about sexually transmitted diseases, one of which was AIDS. AIDS and ITP are CLEARLY two different types of disorders. ITP is not contagious or an STD. Everyone knew I had ITP and like most kids when you learn something new, the first thing you want to do is see if you can connect it to something you already know. So later that day during lunch, all the seventh-graders were outside. I was sitting with my girls at a table just talking about all the drama that was happening. That's when this guy walked over and says, "Mhorgan, we didn't know that you had AIDS." At that point all of my friends and I looked at each other trying to figure out who he was talking to. I was like, "What do you mean I have AIDS?" He explained that in class we learned about the diseases and stuff, so he knew I had a blood disorder and figured it was AIDS. At that point everybody was really confused, and I asked him who all thought I had AIDS. That's when he said everybody. "That's why we kept looking at you and talking, but I just wanted to come and ask you how it feels to have it."

At that point I was thinking: "How stupid and idiotic could someone be?" My friends and I were so outraged by this rumor we just went over to the boys' table and started yelling at them. My friends were rolling their necks, pointing their fingers with the other hand on their hips, and just going in on them. I finally realized technically it wasn't their fault, and I went back to the table and sat down.

I never felt so humiliated and embarrassed until that moment. Everybody was looking at me and I felt like I was under the spotlight. Before I could even stop them, the tears were just rolling down my face, and I had my head down because I was hurt. I just couldn't understand. I didn't even want to at that moment. That's when my principal came outside because even though I wasn't paying it any attention, my friends and the boys were still going back and forth. The principal broke it up and called everyone into his office. By the time I got into the office my parents were already there. I honestly didn't want to talk at that point; I just wanted to go home. Of course that wasn't going to happen, and whether I liked it or not I was going to have to sit there and listen to this long lecture about what I should've done instead of acting on my emotions. So, I walked in the office, sat down, and tried my best to look like I cared what they discussed.

One thing my principal said that really stuck out to me was, "Every situation doesn't call for a reaction." Sometimes it's best to just sit there and let people assume things rather than entertain it. He said, "Mhorgan, you're better than this, and we all know you don't have AIDS; so don't even get worked up about it. We called all the students in the cafeteria and explained to them that you do not have AIDS, and that your disorder is different and by no means contagious. We're sorry this happened, but sometimes when people don't understand something they would rather assume than ask or do the research to learn more."

This event was really a lesson for me. It taught me why it's so important to educate people about the different disorders and things in life and help them become more aware. It really just proved my point that kids need to be educated on these things as well so they at least know how to handle situations. That day I learned that instead of getting mad or upset, all I had to do was simply take a deep breath, calm down and explain to them what I had, and how it affected me and made me feel. Even though I think assuming was ridiculous, I have learned it wasn't their fault because they simply didn't know any better.

I HAVE ITP, BUT ITP DOESN'T HAVE ME

EPILOGUE

There are a lot of things every sick person might want or even wish for.

But one thing a lot of us might wish for but can't actually have is hope. Even though a lot of us want it, few of us allow ourselves to receive it.

We HOPE that one day things will get better. We HOPE that eventually we'll have a day when our pain will finally fade away or even be a zero on the silly little scale of 1-10 that we constantly use to describe the pain the doctors. We HOPE that one day maybe we'll be able to wake up and things go back to what they were or receive a little taste of what being "normal" used to be.

If you ask me if I feel "sick," I'm not going to use the term sick. Let's say imperfect or chronically ill people, especially the younger ones like me, are some of the best people you'll ever meet. Of course, everyone is great too, but when you've been diagnosed with a disorder or you're chronically ill, you take on a whole new perspective of life. To be real, it's the simple things people take for granted that you start to be thankful for and appreciate more. Simply because you can look at how far you've come, and see where you were at one point in your life, and realize no matter who you are, what you have, your life can literally take a dramatic turn at any point in time.

Every second, every minute of each day becomes more and more precious because you realize to embrace everything around you, and cherish all the moments, both good and bad. You're not really sure what tomorrow might bring, but you're not scared to die because you've already come so close to it a few times.

You know, it's not important to dwell on or focus on the little things because you have better, more important things to do. I can't tell you how many times I thought being "normal" would fix all my problems or how I never wanted to have a blood disorder or be sick, and I thought not having ITP would be much easier. However, the older I have become the more I have learned to appreciate my life so much more as the teenage girl that had ITP, who had to learn how to overcome those obstacles in life and still keep going more than I ever could have as a normal teenage girl who just wanted to fit in.

Yes, there were days that ITP made me feel weak, but having ITP overall has made me stronger. It truly gave me knowledge, wisdom, and so much more about life as it ate away at my very own.

Being diagnosed with ITP was the greatest blessing in disguise for me. ITP is so much more than having an illness. It's literally having your entire life taken out of your control, and then making that decision to simply fight for it back. For me, and many others, that fight will never end, but the moment YOU give up, you're giving up your chance to LIVE life to the absolute fullest. Your chance to be able to say: yes, you were diagnosed with something but you REFUSED to let that be the end for you. AND you NEVER gave up.

That's why I can say, "Yes, I have ITP, but IT DOES NOT   HAVE   ME

ABOUT THE AUTHOR

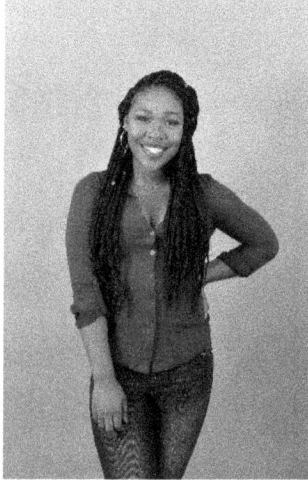

Mhorgan Stephens is currently 17 years old. She was born on August 22, 1999, in Fort Polk, Louisiana. She has two sisters, Jassmon and Zyion Stephens, and is the middle child. Some hobbies Mhorgan enjoys are shopping, cooking, babysitting and spending time with family. She is currently in FBLA, which stands for Future Business Leaders of America, and won first place in district and for the state of South Carolina in public speaking. She is very involved in community service and giving back to others. Along with her foundation for kids with blood disorders, Mhorgan also has her own foundation called Miss Phenomenal, which is a pageant for girls with special needs and disabilities. Her dream in the future is to become a pediatric hematologist and help kids just like her. This is Mhorgan's first book but will certainly not be her last.